57 Quick Juicing Solutions for Diarrhea and Stomach Aches:

Organic Juice Recipes That Will Help You Recover Quickly

By

Joe Correa CSN

COPYRIGHT

© 2018 Live Stronger Faster Inc.

This publication is designed to provide accurate and authoritative information in regard to the subject matter covered. It is sold with the understanding that neither the author nor the publisher is engaged in rendering medical advice. If medical advice or assistance is needed, consult with a doctor. This book is considered a guide and should not be used in any way detrimental to your health. Consult with a physician before starting this nutritional plan to make sure it's right for you.

ACKNOWLEDGEMENTS

This book is dedicated to my friends and family that have had mild or serious illnesses so that you may find a solution and make the necessary changes in your life.

57 Quick Juicing Solutions for Diarrhea and Stomach Aches:

Organic Juice Recipes That Will Help You Recover Quickly

By

Joe Correa CSN

CONTENTS

ABOUT THE AUTHOR

After years of Research, I honestly believe in the positive effects that proper nutrition can have over the body and mind. My knowledge and experience has helped me live healthier throughout the years and which I have shared with family and friends. The more you know about eating and drinking healthier, the sooner you will want to change your life and eating habits.

Nutrition is a key part in the process of being healthy and living longer so get started today. The first step is the most important and the most significant.

INTRODUCTION

57 Quick Juicing Solutions for Diarrhea and Stomach Aches: Organic Juice Recipes That Will Help You Recover Quickly

By Joe Correa CSN

Frequent loose and watery stools caused by an increased secretion of fluid into the intestine and reduced absorption of fluid from the intestine is known as diarrhea. This condition usually lasts for just a couple of days and goes away on its own. In some more severe cases, diarrhea can last up to 3-4 weeks and sometimes even develop into a chronic disease.

Diarrhea is a medical condition that can affect most of the population, regardless of age or sex. Most adults in the United States have diarrhea at least once a year. Children, on the other hand, tend to suffer from diarrhea more often, on average twice per year.

Diarrhea can be caused by different factors. The most common include:

- Contaminated food or water
- Different viruses
- Some parasites found in food or water

- Various medicines
- Problems with digestion of certain foods and food intolerances (like lactose intolerance)
- Diseases of the digestive tract
- Irritable bowel syndrome

Diarrhea is often followed by common and recognizable symptoms like sharp pain and cramps in the abdomen, an urgent and uncontrollable need to use the bathroom, and liquid stools. Naturally, this condition can cause dehydration which can be quite dangerous, especially for newborns and older people. In this case, urgent medical attention is needed.

When it comes to treatment, in most cases, diarrhea goes away on its own. However, rehydration is extremely important in order to replace lost fluids in the body. People suffering from diarrhea are often advised to drink plenty of fruit and vegetable juices, sodas without caffeine, and broths. In more serious cases, oral rehydration solutions are often prescribed.

This book contains some fantastic juice recipes that were carefully chosen to help eliminate diarrhea and rehydrate the entire body. These juices are based on fresh fruits and vegetables that have the ability to clean the entire digestive tract and help your body heal within a couple of days. Furthermore, these juices take only a couple of minutes to prepare which means you can enjoy them all day long.

Give these juices a try and see which ones you like the most!

COMMITMENT

In order to improve my condition, I *(your name)*, commit to eating more of these foods on a daily basis and to exercise at least 30 minutes daily:

- Berries (especially blueberries), peaches, cherries, apples, apricots, oranges, lemon juice, grapefruit, tangerines, mandarins, pears, etc.
- Broccoli, spinach, collard greens, sweet potatoes, avocado, artichoke, baby corn, carrots, celery, cauliflower, onions, etc.
- Whole grains, steel-cut oats, oatmeal, quinoa, barley, etc.
- Black beans, red bean beans, garbanzo beans, lentils, etc.
- Nuts and seeds including: walnuts, cashews, flaxseeds, sesame seeds, etc.
- Fish
- 8 – 10 glasses of water

Sign here

X_____

57 QUICK JUICING SOLUTIONS FOR DIARRHEA AND STOMACH ACHES

1.   Banana Blueberry Juice

Ingredients:

2 large bananas, peeled

1 cup blueberries, fresh

1 medium-sized radish, sliced

1 tbsp fresh mint, chopped

1 cup cauliflower, chopped

¼ cup water

Preparation:

Peel the bananas and cut into thin slices. Set aside.

Wash the blueberries under cold running water. Drain and set aside.

Wash the radish and trim off the green parts. Cut into small pieces and set aside.

Trim off the outer leaves of cauliflower. Wash it and cut into small pieces. Reserve the rest in the refrigerator.

Now, combine bananas, blueberries, radish, cauliflower and mint in a juicer. Process until juiced.

Transfer to serving glasses and stir in the coconut water.

Add some ice and serve.

Nutritional information per serving: Kcal: 232, Protein: 5.2g, Carbs: 98.9g, Fats: 1.7g

2. Artichoke Brussels Sprout Juice

Ingredients:

1 large artichoke, chopped

1 cup Brussels sprouts, chopped

1 cup mustard greens, chopped

1 medium-sized Red Delicious apple, peeled and cored

½ tsp cinnamon, freshly ground

½ cup coconut water, unsweetened

1 tsp honey

Preparation:

Trim off the outer leave of the artichoke using a sharp knife. Rinse well and cut into small pieces. Set aside.

Rinse the Brussels sprouts and trim off the outer layers. Chop into small pieces and set aside.

Place the mustard greens in a large colander and rinse under running water. Torn into small pieces and set aside.

Wash the apple and remove the core. Cut into bite-sized pieces and set aside.

Now, place artichoke, Brussels sprouts, mustard greens, and apple in a juicer. Process until juiced.

Transfer to serving glasses and stir in the cinnamon, coconut water, and honey.

Add some ice and serve immediately.

Nutritional information per serving: Kcal: 195, Protein: 13.7g, Carbs: 63.4g, Fats: 1.3g

3.   Beet Juice

Ingredients:

1 cup beets, trimmed

1 cup beet greens, chopped

1 cup cauliflower, chopped

1 cup parsnips, chopped

2 tbsp fresh mint, finely chopped

Preparation:

Wash the beets and trim off the green parts. Cut into small pieces. Chop the greens and set aside.

Wash the parsnips and cut into thick slices. Set aside.

Trim off the outer leaves of a cauliflower. Wash it and chop into small pieces. Set aside.

Now, combine beets, beet greens, cauliflower, and parsnips in a juicer. Process until juiced.

Transfer to serving glasses and refrigerate for 10 minutes. Garnish with fresh mint before serving.

Nutritional information per serving: Kcal: 167, Protein: 9.8g, Carbs: 52.8g, Fats: 1.6g

4.   Honeycrisp Chia Juice

Ingredients:

1 small Honeycrisp apple, cored

1 cup cucumber, sliced

½ red bell pepper, seeded

½ yellow bell pepper, seeded

3 tbsp chia seeds

Preparation:

Peel the cucumber and cut into thin slices. Fill the measuring cup and reserve the rest in the refrigerator.

Rinse peppers and cut in half. Remove the seeds and chop one-half into small pieces. Place in a bowl. Reserve the rest in the refrigerator.

Wash the apple and remove the core. Cut into bite-sized pieces and set aside.

Now, combine cucumber, bell peppers, and apple in a juicer. Transfer to serving glasses and stir in the chia seeds.

Refrigerate for 15 minutes before serving.

Enjoy!

Nutritional information per serving: Kcal: 136, Protein: 4.3g, Carbs: 31.2g, Fats: 6.1g

5.   Banana Apricot Juice

Ingredients:

1 large banana, chunked

1 large apricot, pitted

1 cup cauliflower florets, chopped

1 cup broccoli, chopped

Preparation:

Peel the banana and cut into small chunks. Set aside.

Wash the apricot and cut in half. Remove the pit and cut into small pieces. Set aside.

Rinse the cauliflower florets under running water using a colander. Drain and set aside.

Place the broccoli in a colander and wash under cold running water. Chop into small pieces and set aside.

Combine banana, apricot, grapefruit, and broccoli in a juicer. Transfer to serving glasses and refrigerate for 30 minutes before serving.

Nutritional information per serving: Kcal: 229, Protein: 6.5g, Carbs: 67.2g, Fats: 1.3g

6.   Apple Carrot Juice

Ingredients:

1 large Golden Delicious apple, peeled and cored

1 large carrot, sliced

½ cup of butternut squash, chopped

1 tbsp of fresh mint, finely chopped

1 large banana, sliced

¼ tsp ginger, ground

Preparation:

Wash the apple and remove the core. Cut into bite-sized pieces and set aside.

Wash the carrot and cut into small slices. Set aside.

Peel the butternut squash and remove the seeds using a spoon. Cut into small cubes and reserve the rest of the squash for some other recipe. Wrap in a plastic foil and refrigerate.

Peel the banana and cut into thin slices. Set aside.

Now, combine apple carrot, butternut squash, and banana in a juicer. Process until juiced.

Transfer to serving glasses and stir in the mint for some extra taste.

Add some ice and serve.

Nutritional information per serving: Kcal: 372, Protein: 5.5g, Carbs: 73.4g, Fats: 1.4g

7.   Leek Brussels Sprout Juice

Ingredients:

2 whole leeks, chopped

1 cup of Brussels sprouts, chopped

1 cup of parsley, chopped

A handful of spinach, chopped

½ cup of water

Preparation:

Wash the leeks and chop into small pieces. Set aside.

Wash the Brussels sprouts and trim off the outer leaves. Cut in half and set aside.

Wash the parsley in a colander under cold running water and set aside.

Wash the spinach thoroughly and set aside.

Combine leeks, Brussels sprouts, parsley, and spinach in a juicer. Transfer to serving glasses and stir in the water.

Refrigerate for 10 minutes before serving.

Nutritional information per serving: Kcal: 120, Protein: 6.4g, Carbs: 46.2g, Fats: 1.8g

8.   Cabbage Carrot Juice

Ingredients:

2 cups of green cabbage, shredded

1 cup of carrots, chopped

2 small Granny Smith's apples, core

1 large banana, peeled

1 tbsp of honey, raw

Preparation:

Wash the cabbage thoroughly and roughly chop it using hands. Set aside.

Wash the carrots and cut into small pieces. Set aside.

Peel the apples and cut in half. Remove the core and cut into bite-sized pieces. Set aside.

Peel the banana and cut into thin slices. Set aside.

Now, combine cabbage, carrots, apples, and banana in a juicer. Process until juiced.

Transfer to serving glasses and stir in the honey.

Add some ice cubes and serve immediately.

Nutritional information per serving: Kcal: 219, Protein: 6.9g, Carbs: 69g, Fats: 1.5g

9.   Maple Peach Juice

Ingredients:

1 large peach, peeled

1 cup parsnip, sliced

½ cup strawberries, chopped

3 cups lettuce, torn

1 tsp maple syrup

Preparation:

Rinse the peach and cut in half. Remove the pit and cut into bite-sized pieces. Set aside.

Wash and peel the parsnips. Cut into thick slices and set aside.

Rinse the strawberries and remove the stems. Cut into halves and set aside.

Rinse the lettuce thoroughly using a colander. Torn into small pieces and set aside.

Now, combine peach, parsnips, strawberries, and lettuce in a juicer. Process until juiced. Transfer to serving glasses and stir in the maple syrup.

Add some ice and serve immediately.

Nutritional information per serving: Kcal: 186, Protein: 5.4g, Carbs: 63.7g, Fats: 1.1g

10.   Mango Banana Juice

Ingredients:

1 large mango

1 large banana, peeled

1 large guava, peeled

¼ cup coconut water

Preparation:

Peel the mango and cut into small chunks. Set aside.

Peel the banana and cut into thin slices. Set aside.

Wash the guava and cut into chunks. If you are using large fruit, reserve the rest for some other recipe in a refrigerator. Set aside.

Now, combine mango, banana, and guava in a juicer. Transfer to serving glasses and stir in the coconut water.

Add few ice cubes and serve immediately.

Enjoy!

Nutritional information per serving: Kcal: 295, Protein: 4.4g, Carbs: 88.9g, Fats: 1.8g

11.   Cabbage Apple Juice

Ingredients:

1 cup of green cabbage, chopped

1 large Fuji apple, cored

1 cup of pumpkin, seeded and peeled

1 large banana, peeled

¼ tsp ginger powder

Preparation:

Rinse the cabbage thoroughly using a colander. Chop into small pieces and set aside.

Wash the apple and remove the core. Cut into bite-sized pieces and set aside.

Peel the pumpkin and cut in half. Scoop out the seeds using a spoon. Cut one large wedge and peel it. Cut into small chunks and set aside.

Peel the banana and cut into thin slices. Set aside.

Now, combine cabbage, apple, pumpkin, and banana in a juicer. Transfer to serving glasses and add few ice cubes.

Refrigerate for 10-15 minutes before serving.

Nutritional information per serving: Kcal: 228, Protein: 5.4g, Carbs: 69.3g, Fats: 1.5g

12.   Radish Mint Juice

Ingredients:

1 medium-sized radish, chopped

1 tbsp of fresh mint, chopped

1 cup of cantaloupe, diced

1 cup of beet greens, chopped

1 cup of cauliflower, chopped

Preparation:

Wash the radish and trim off the green parts. Cut into small chunks and set aside.

Soak the mint leaves in water. Let it stand for 2 minutes.

Trim off the outer leaves of cauliflower. Wash it and cut into small pieces. Reserve the rest in the refrigerator.

Cut the cantaloupe in half. Scoop out the seeds and flesh. Cut two wedges and peel them. Chop into chunks and set aside. Reserve the rest of the cantaloupe in a refrigerator.

Wash the beet greens and torn with hands. Set aside.

Now, combine cantaloupe, beet greens, radish, cauliflower and mint in a juicer. Process until juiced.

Transfer to serving glasses and add some ice before serving.

Nutritional information per serving: Kcal: 123, Protein: 8.1g, Carbs: 37.7g, Fats: 1.1g

13.   Grape Broccoli Juice

Ingredients:

½ cup of black grapes

1 cup broccoli, chopped

1 medium-sized pear, roughly chopped

1 cup of spinach, torn

1 small ginger root slice, peeled

Preparation:

Wash the pear and remove the core. Cut into small pieces and set aside.

Rinse the broccoli and cut into small pieces. Fill the measuring cup and reserve the rest in the refrigerator.

Wash the grapes in a colander under cold running water and set aside.

Wash the spinach thoroughly and torn with hands. Set aside.

Peel the ginger slice and set aside.

Combine pear, grapes, oranges, spinach, and ginger in a juicer and process until juiced.

Transfer to serving glasses and refrigerate for 15 minutes before serving.

Enjoy!

Nutritional information per serving: Kcal: 217, Protein: 6.2g, Carbs: 75.4g, Fats: 1.2g

14. Spinach Coconut Juice

Ingredients:

2 cups fresh spinach

½ cup of coconut water, unsweetened

1 cup of broccoli, chopped

1 tbsp of honey, raw

A few mint leaves

Preparation:

Wash the broccoli and trim off the outer leaves. Set aside.

Rinse the spinach thoroughly under running water. Drain and torn with hands. Set aside.

Now, combine broccoli and spinach in a juicer. Process until juiced.

Transfer to serving glasses and stir in the honey and garnish with mint leaves.

Add some ice and serve immediately.

Nutritional information per serving: Kcal: 171, Protein: 14.8g, Carbs: 54.5g, Fats: 2.17g

15.   Watermelon Spinach Juice

Ingredients:

2 cups watermelon, roughly chopped

2 cups spinach, chopped

2 cups fresh strawberries, chopped

1 medium-sized banana, peeled

½ tsp of cinnamon, ground

1 tsp of honey, raw

Preparation:

Cut the watermelon in half. Cut two large wedges and peel. Cut into small chunks and remove the seeds. Fill the measuring cups and reserve the rest for later.

Rinse the spinach thoroughly and torn with hands. Set aside.

Rinse the strawberries under cold running water and remove the stems. Chop into small pieces and set aside.

Peel the banana and cut into small chunks. Set aside.

Now, combine strawberries, melon, spinach, and banana in a juicer. Process until juiced. Transfer to serving glasses and stir in the honey and cinnamon.

Refrigerate for 10 minutes before serving minutes.

Nutritional information per serving: Kcal: 349, Protein: 7.6g, Carbs: 104.9g, Fats: 3.2g

16.   Blueberry Coconut Juice

Ingredients:

2 cups strawberries, chopped

1 cup blueberries

½ cup coconut water, unsweetened

1 tsp agave nectar

Preparation:

Combine blueberries and strawberries in a colander and wash under cold running water. Set aside.

Peel the orange and divide into wedges. Use about half of the wedges and reserve the rest for some other juice.

Combine blueberries and strawberries in a juicer. Transfer to serving glasses and stir in the coconut water and agave nectar.

Add some ice or refrigerate before serving.

Nutritional information per serving: Kcal: 246, Protein: 4.7g, Carbs: 74.2g, Fats: 1.7g

17.   Sweet Apple Banana Juice

Ingredients:

2 large Granny Smith apples, cored and chopped

1 large banana, peeled

1 tsp of honey, raw

½ tsp of ginger, freshly ground

Preparation:

Wash the apples and remove the core. Chop into bite-sized pieces and set aside.

Peel the banana and cut into thin slices. Set aside.

Now, combine apples and banana in a juicer. Transfer to serving glasses and stir in the honey and ginger.

Refrigerate or add some ice and serve.

Enjoy!

Nutritional information per serving: Kcal: 299, Protein: 3.7g, Carbs: 88g, Fats: 1.1g

18.   Cucumber Fuji Juice

Ingredients:

3 large cucumbers, peeled

1 Fuji apple, peeled

1 tsp peppermint extract

1 tbsp fresh mint, chopped

Preparation:

Wash the cucumbers and cut into thick slices. Set aside.

Peel the apple and remove the core. Cut into bite-sized pieces and set aside.

Now, combine cucumber and apple in a juicer and process until juiced. Transfer to serving glasses and stir in the peppermint extract.

Add some ice cubes and serve immediately.

Nutritional information per serving: Kcal: 204, Protein: 7.7g, Carbs: 59g, Fats: 1.3g

19.   Banana Raspberry Juice

Ingredients:

1 large banana, peeled

1 cup raspberries, fresh

1 cup butternut squash, chopped

½ cup coconut water

1 tsp honey

Preparation:

Peel the banana and cut into chunks. Set aside.

Wash the raspberries under cold running water. Drain and set aside.

Peel the butternut squash and remove the seeds using a spoon. Cut into small cubes and reserve the rest of the squash for some other recipe. Wrap in a plastic foil and refrigerate.

Now, combine banana, raspberries, and butternut squash in a juicer. Transfer to serving glasses and stir in the coconut water and honey.

Add some ice and serve immediately.

Enjoy!

Nutritional information per serving: Kcal: 197, Protein: 4.7g, Carbs: 68g, Fats: 1.3g

20.   Kale Cranberry Juice

Ingredients:

1 cup fresh kale, torn

1 cup cranberries

1 small Honeycrisp apple, cored

¼ cup coconut water

Preparation:

Peel the kiwis and cut lengthwise in half. Set aside.

Rinse the kale thoroughly and into small pieces. Fill the measuring cup and set aside.

Wash the cranberries under cold running water. Drain and set aside.

Now, combine kale, cranberries, and apple in a juicer. Transfer to serving glasses and stir in the coconut water.

Add some ice and serve immediately.

Nutritional information per serving: Kcal: 153, Protein: 5.6g, Carbs: 48.4g, Fats: 1.8g

21.   Blackberry Banana Juice

Ingredients:

2 cups blackberries

1 large banana, peeled

2 cups spinach, chopped

2 cups beet greens, chopped

¼ cup water

Preparation:

Rinse the blackberries under cold running water. Drain and set aside.

Peel the banana and cut into chunks. Set aside.

Combine spinach and beet greens in a colander and wash thoroughly. Chop into small pieces and set aside.

Now, combine blackberries, banana, spinach, and beet greens in a juicer. Process until juiced.

Transfer to serving glasses and add some ice cubes before serving.

Enjoy!

Nutritional information per serving: Kcal: 183, Protein: 7.8g, Carbs: 63.1g, Fats: 1.2g

22.　　Blackberry Turnip Juice

Ingredients:

1 cup of plums, halved

1 cup of fresh blackberries

1 cup of turnip greens, chopped

½ tsp of ginger, ginger

½ cup of water

Preparation:

Rinse the blackberries under cold running water using a colander. Drain and set aside.

Rinse the turnip greens and torn into small pieces. Set aside.

Wash the plums and cut in half. Remove the pits and set aside.

Now, combine plums, blackberries, and turnip greens in a juicer and process until juiced.

Transfer to serving glasses and stir in the ginger and water.

Refrigerate for 5 minutes before serving.

Enjoy!

Nutritional information per serving: Kcal: 141, Protein: 4.2g, Carbs: 40.3g, Fats: 1.4g

23.   Radish Beet Juice

Ingredients:

2 cups radishes, chopped

1 cup of beet greens, torn

1 cup of watercress, chopped

1 tbsp of honey, raw

Preparation:

Wash the radishes and trim off the green parts. Cut into small pieces and set aside.

Place the beet greens and watercress in a large colander. Rinse under cold running water and torn into small pieces.

Now, combine radishes, beet greens, and watercress in a juicer and process until juiced.

Transfer to serving glasses and add some ice before serving.

Enjoy!

Nutritional information per serving: Kcal: 147, Protein: 5.3g, Carbs: 50g, Fats: 0.8g

24.   Peach Spinach Juice

Ingredients:

1 large peach, chopped

1 cup spinach, torn

2 large Red Delicious apples, peeled and cored

1 large carrot, sliced

¼ cup water

Preparation:

Wash the peach and cut in half. Remove the pit and chop into small pieces. Set aside.

Rinse the spinach thoroughly and torn with hands. Set aside.

Wash the apples and remove the core. Cut into thin slices and set aside.

Wash the carrot and cut into thick slices. Set aside.

Now, combine apples, peach, spinach, and carrot in a juicer and process until juiced.

Transfer to serving glasses and refrigerate for 10 minutes before serving.

Nutritional information per serving: Kcal: 297, Protein: 5.5g, Carbs: 87.5g, Fats: 1.5g

25.   Broccoli Coconut Juice

Ingredients:

2 cups raw broccoli, chopped

½ cup coconut water

1 cup fresh raspberries

2 large cucumbers, peeled

1 tbsp honey

Preparation:

Wash the raspberries under cold running water. Drain and set aside.

Wash the broccoli and cut into small pieces. Set aside.

Wash and peel the cucumbers. Cut into thick slices and set aside.

Combine broccoli, cucumber, and raspberries in a juicer and process until juiced.

Transfer to serving glasses and stir in the coconut water and honey.

Add some ice and serve.

Nutritional information per serving: Kcal: 192, Protein: 10.9g, Carbs: 56g, Fats: 2.2g

26.   Leek Brussels Sprout Juice

Ingredients:

1 whole leek, chopped

1 cup of Brussels sprouts, chopped

1 large green apple, peeled and seeds removed

2 cups of mustard greens, chopped

1 medium-sized zucchini, peeled

1 cup of parsnip, sliced

Preparation:

Wash the leek and cut into small pieces. Set aside.

Wash the Brussels sprouts and trim off the outer leaves. Set aside.

Wash the apple and remove the core. Cut into bite-sized pieces and set aside.

Wash the mustard greens and torn with hands. Set aside.

Wash the zucchini and cut in half. Scoop out the seeds using a spoon. Cut into small chunks and set aside.

Wash the parsnips and cut into thick slices. Set aside.

Now, combine leek, Brussels sprouts, apple, mustard greens, zucchini and parsnips in a juicer.

Transfer to serving glasses and refrigerate for 5 minutes before serving.

Nutritional information per serving: Kcal: 284, Protein: 12.3g, Carbs: 83.7g, Fats: 2.4g

27.   Cabbage Apple Juice

Ingredients:

1 cup of purple cabbage, torn

1 Granny Smith's apple, cored

1 cup of red leaf lettuce, torn

1 cup of papaya, chopped

¼ cup coconut water

1 tsp maple syrup

Preparation:

Combine lettuce and cabbage in a large colander. Rinse under cold running water. Chop into small pieces and set aside.

Peel the papaya and cut lengthwise in half. Scoop out the black seeds and flesh using a spoon. Cut into small chunks and set aside.

Now, combine cabbage, apple, lettuce, and papaya in a juicer. Process until juiced.

Transfer to serving glasses and stir in the coconut water and maple syrup.

Add some ice and serve immediately.

Nutritional information per serving: Kcal: 201, Protein: 7g, Carbs: 61.7g, Fats: 1.7g

28.   Broccoli Goji Juice

Ingredients:

1 cup broccoli, pre-cooked

1 cup Goji berries

1 large orange, peeled

1 large cucumber, peeled

2 tsp maple syrup

Preparation:

Wash the broccoli and chop into small pieces. Set aside.

Place the goji berries in a medium bowl. Add 1 cup of water and soak for 30 minutes.

Wash the cucumber and cut into thick slices. Set aside.

Now, combine broccoli, goji berries, and cucumber in a juicer. Process until juiced.

Transfer to serving glasses and stir in the honey.

Add some ice and serve!

Nutritional information per serving: Kcal: 193, Protein: 9.4g, Carbs: 66g, Fats: 1.7g

29.   Vanilla Banana Juice

Ingredients:

1 large banana, sliced

1 large Fuji Apple, cored

1 tsp pure vanilla extract, sugar-free

¼ cup coconut water

Preparation:

Peel the banana and cut into thin slices. Set aside.

Rinse the apple and remove the core. Cut into bite-sized pieces and set aside.

Now, combine banana and apple in a juicer and process until juiced.

Transfer to a serving glass and stir in the vanilla extract and coconut water.

Refrigerate for 10 minutes before serving.

Nutritional information per serving: Kcal: 292, Protein: 6.9g, Carbs: 96g, Fats: 2g

30.   Banana Apple Juice

Ingredients:

1 cup banana, sliced

1 small apple, peeled and seeds removed

1 cup fresh mint leaves, finely chopped

¼ tsp of nutmeg, ground

¼ tsp cinnamon, ground

1 tbsp maple syrup

¼ cup water

Preparation:

Peel the banana and cut into thin slices. Fill the measuring cup and reserve the rest in the refrigerator.

Rinse the apple and remove the core. Cut into bite-sized pieces and set aside.

Now, combine banana, apple and mint in a juicer. Transfer to a serving glasses and stir in the nutmeg, cinnamon, maple syrup, and water

Garnish with some extra mint leaves and refrigerate before serving.

Add some ice and serve immediately.

Nutritional information per serving: Kcal: 141, Protein: 1.5g, Carbs: 41.2g, Fats: 0.4g

31.   Banana Blueberry Juice

Ingredients:

1 large banana, sliced

1 cup blueberries

1 tsp of flaxseeds

½ cup celery, chopped

1 tbsp of honey

Preparation:

Peel the banana and cut into small chunks. Set aside.

Rinse the blueberries under running water. Drain and set aside.

Rinse the celery and chop into bite-sized pieces. Set aside.

Now, combine banana blueberries, and celery in a juicer. Transfer to serving glasses and stir in the flaxseeds and honey.

Add few ice cubes before serving.

Enjoy!

Nutritional information per serving: Kcal: 177, Protein: 6.5g, Carbs: 44.6g, Fats: 2.6g

32.   Kale Strawberry Juice

Ingredients:

1 cup of fresh kale, torn

1 cup of strawberries, fresh

½ tsp of ginger, ground

¼ cup coconut water

Preparation:

Rinse the kale thoroughly under running water. Chop into small pieces and set aside.

Wash the strawberries and remove the stems. Chop into small pieces and set aside.

Combine kale and strawberries in a juicer and process until juiced.

Transfer to serving glasses and stir in the ginger and coconut water. Add some ice cubes before serving.

Enjoy!

Nutritional information per serving: Kcal: 120, Protein: 5.9g, Carbs: 38.6g, Fats: 1.8g

33.   Apple Mango Juice

Ingredients:

1 medium-sized Granny Smith's apple, chopped

1 cup of mango chunks

1 cup of guava chunks

1 tbsp of fresh mint leaves

½ cup of coconut water

Preparation:

Wash the apple and cut in half. Remove the core and cut into bite-sized pieces. Set aside.

Peel the mango and cut into small chunks. Set aside.

Wash the guava and cut into chunks. If you are using large fruit, reserve the rest for some other recipe in a refrigerator.

Now, combine apple, mango, and guava in a juicer. Process until juiced.

Transfer to serving glasses and stir in the coconut water.

Garnish with some mint leaves and add some ice before serving.

Enjoy!

Nutritional information per serving: Kcal: 187, Protein: 3.6g, Carbs: 54.2g, Fats: 1.3g

34.   Carrot Parsnip Juice

Ingredients:

3 large carrots, sliced

1 cup of parsnips, sliced

2 large Fuji apples, peeled and cored

1 tbsp fresh basil, finely chopped

¼ cup of water

Preparation:

Wash the apples and cut into halves. Remove the core and cut into bite-sized pieces. Set aside.

Wash the carrots and parsnips and cut into thick slices. Set aside.

Now, combine carrots, parsnips, and apples in a juicer and process until juiced.

Transfer to serving glasses and stir in the water. Garnish with basil leaves and refrigerate before serving.

Enjoy!

Nutritional information per serving: Kcal: 332, Protein: 5.4g, Carbs: 100g, Fats: 1.6g

35.   Banana Apricot Juice

Ingredients:

1 large banana, sliced

1 cup apricots, chopped

1 large cucumber, sliced

1 cup fresh spinach, torn

½ cup of raw broccoli, chopped

½ cup of pure coconut water

Preparation:

Peel the banana and cut into thin slices. Set aside.

Wash the apricots and cut in half. Remove the pit and chop into chunks. Set aside.

Wash the cucumber and chop into thick slices. Set aside.

Combine spinach and broccoli in a colander and wash under cold running water. Drain and roughly chop. Set aside.

Now, combine banana, apricots, cucumber, spinach, and broccoli in a juicer. Process until juiced. Transfer to serving glasses and stir in the coconut water.

Add some ice and serve immediately.

Nutritional information per serving: Kcal: 218, Protein: 10g, Carbs: 64g, Fats: 1.9g

36.   Mint Cranberry Juice

Ingredients:

1 tbsp fresh mint, finely chopped

1 cup fresh cranberries

2 cups cherries, pitted

1 cup leek, chopped

1 tbsp maple syrup

Preparation:

Wash the cranberries under cold running water and set aside.

Wash the cherries under cold running water. Drain and cut in half. Remove the pits and set aside.

Wash the leek and cut into small pieces. Set aside.

Combine cherries, leek, cranberries, and mint in a juicer and process until juiced.

Transfer to serving glasses and stir in the honey.

Add some ice and serve!

Nutritional information per serving: Kcal: 248, Protein: 5g, Carbs: 75.5g, Fats: 1g

37.   Raspberry Cabbage Juice

Ingredients:

1 cup raspberries

1 cup purple cabbage, torn

1 cup papaya, chopped

1 tsp ginger, ground

1 tsp honey

Preparation:

Rinse the raspberries under cold running water. Drain and set aside.

Rinse the cabbage thoroughly and torn with hands. Set aside.

Peel the papaya and cut lengthwise in half. Scoop out the black seeds and flesh using a spoon. Cut into small chunks and set aside.

Combine raspberries, cabbage, and papaya in a juicer and process until juiced.

Transfer to serving glasses and stir in the ginger and honey.

Add some ice cubes and serve immediately.

Nutritional information per serving: Kcal: 172, Protein: 4.3g, Carbs: 54.2g, Fats: 0.7g

38. Radish Swiss Chard Juice

Ingredients:

1 large radish, chopped

1 cup Swiss chard, torn

1 large honeydew melon wedge

1 cup asparagus, chopped

1 cup avocado, chopped

¼ cup coconut water

Preparation:

Wash the radish and trim off the green parts. Cut into small pieces and set aside.

Wash the chard thoroughly and torn with hands. Set aside.

Cut the honeydew melon lengthwise in half. Scoop out the seeds using a spoon. Cut the large wedges and peel them. Cut into small chunks and place in a bowl. Wrap the rest of the melon in a plastic foil and refrigerate.

Wash the asparagus and trim off the woody ends. Set aside.

Peel the avocado and cut in half. Remove the pit and cut into chunks. Set aside.

Now, combine radish, chard, melon, asparagus, and avocado in a juicer. Process until juiced.

Transfer to serving glasses and refrigerate 10 minutes before serving.

Nutritional information per serving: Kcal: 275, Protein: 8g, Carbs: 35.2g, Fats: 21.9g

39.   Celery Beet Juice

Ingredients:

1 cup of celery, chopped

1 cup of beets, sliced

1 cup of beet greens, chopped

1 cup of crookneck squash, sliced

1 cup of pomegranate seeds

1 tbsp of honey

Preparation:

Wash the celery and cut into small pieces. Set aside.

Wash the beets and trim off the green parts. Cut into bite-sized pieces and set aside.

Use the trimmed beet greens and roughly chop it.

Wash the crookneck squash and cut in half. Scoop out the seeds using a spoon. Cut into small chunks and set aside. Reserve the rest for another juice.

Cut the top of the pomegranate fruit using a sharp knife. Slice down to each of the white membranes inside of the fruit. Pop the seeds into a measuring cup and set aside.

Now, combine celery, beets, beet greens, celery, and pomegranate seeds in a juicer.

Transfer to serving glasses and stir in the honey.

Add some ice and serve immediately.

Nutritional information per serving: Kcal: 132, Protein: 6.4g, Carbs: 48.8g, Fats: 1.8g

40.   Tomato Swiss Chard Juice

Ingredients:

1 large tomato, chopped

1 cup of Swiss chard, chopped

1 cup of asparagus, trimmed

1 cup of Brussels sprouts, trimmed

1 large cucumber, sliced

Preparation:

Wash the tomato and place in a bowl. Cut into quarters and reserve the juice while cutting. Set aside.

Wash the Swiss chard thoroughly under cold running water. Drain and set aside.

Wash the asparagus and trim off the woody ends. Cut into 1-inch pieces and set aside.

Wash the Brussels sprouts and trim off the outer layers. Cut in half and set aside.

Wash the cucumber and cut into thick slices. Set aside.

Now, combine tomato, Swiss chard, asparagus, Brussels sprouts, and cucumber in a juicer. Process until juiced.

Transfer to serving glasses and add some ice before serving.

Nutrition information per serving: Kcal: 109, Protein: 10.1g, Carbs: 32.4g, Fats: 1.2g

41.   Avocado Cucumber Juice

Ingredients:

1 large tomato, chopped

1 cup avocado, chopped

1 large cucumber, sliced

1 cup of fresh basil, chopped

Preparation:

Peel the avocado and cut in half. Remove the pit and cut into chunks. Fill the measuring cup and reserve the rest for some other juice. Keep it in a refrigerator.

Wash the cucumber and cut into thick slices. Set aside.

Wash the tomato and place in a bowl. Cut into quarters and reserve the juice while cutting. Set aside.

Wash the basil thoroughly and roughly chop it. Set aside.

Now, combine tomato, avocado, cucumber, and basil in a juicer and process until juiced.

Transfer to serving glasses and add some ice before serving.

Enjoy!

Nutrition information per serving: Kcal: 240, Protein: 3.1g, Carbs: 75.1g, Fats: 0.9g

42.   Watermelon Mint Juice

Ingredients:

1 cup of watermelon, chopped

1 large banana, sliced

1 large peach, pitted and halved

1 large Fuji apple, cored

3 tbsp of fresh mint, chopped

Preparation:

Cut the watermelon lengthwise. For two cups, you will need about two large wedges. Peel and cut into chunks. Remove the seeds and set aside. Reserve the rest of the melon for some other juices.

Peel the banana and cut into slices. Set aside.

Wash the peach and cut in half. Remove the pit and cut into chunks. Set aside.

Wash the apple and remove the core. Cut into bite-sized pieces and set aside.

Now, combine watermelon, banana, peach, and apple in a juicer and process until juiced.

Transfer to serving glasses and garnish with some fresh mint. Add some ice cubes before serving.

Enjoy!

Nutrition information per serving: Kcal: 269, Protein: 5.3g, Carbs: 78.5g, Fats: 1.3g

43.   Avocado Lettuce Juice

Ingredients:

1 cup of avocado, sliced

3 cups red leaf lettuce, torn

1 large Fuji apple, chopped

½ cup coconut water

1 tsp of liquid honey

Preparation:

Peel the avocado and cut in half. Remove the pit and chop into chunks. Fill the measuring cup and reserve the rest for some other juice. Set aside.

Wash the lettuce thoroughly under cold running water. Torn with hands and set aside.

Wash the apple and remove the core. Cut into bite-sized pieces and set aside.

Now, combine avocado, lettuce, and orange in a juicer and process until juiced.

Transfer to serving glasses and refrigerate for 5 minutes before serving.

Enjoy!

Nutrition information per serving: Kcal: 240, Protein: 4.9g, Carbs: 25.6g, Fats: 21.7g

44.   Broccoli Brussels Sprout Juice

Ingredients:

1 cup of broccoli, chopped

1 cup of Brussels sprouts, chopped

1 cup of carrots, sliced

1 cup of turnip greens, chopped

2 small Honeycrisp apples, chopped

1 tbsp of honey

¼ cup coconut water

Preparation:

Wash the broccoli and cut into small pieces. Set aside.

Wash the Brussels sprouts and trim off the outer layers. Cut in half and set aside.

Wash the carrots and cut into thick slices. Set aside.

Wash the turnip greens thoroughly and torn with hands. Set aside.

Wash the apples and cut into halves. Remove the core and chop into small pieces. Set aside.

Now, combine broccoli, Brussels sprouts, carrots, turnip greens, and apples in a juicer and process until juiced.

Transfer to serving glasses and stir in the honey and coconut water. Add some ice cubes before serving or refrigerate for 5 minutes.

Enjoy!

Nutrition information per serving: Kcal: 367, Protein: 14.47g, Carbs: 116g, Fats: 1.9g

45.   Blackberry Banana Juice

Ingredients:

1 cup of blackberries, fresh

1 large banana, peeled

2 cups watermelon, seeded

½ cup of pure coconut water, unsweetened

1 tbsp of honey

Preparation:

Wash the blackberries under cold running water and set aside.

Peel the banana and cut into thin slices. Set aside.

Cut the watermelon lengthwise. Cut two large wedges and peel them. Cut into chunks and remove the seeds. Set aside.

Now, combine blackberries, banana, and watermelon in a juicer and process until juiced.

Transfer to serving glasses and stir the coconut water and honey.

Refrigerate for 5 minutes before serving.

Enjoy!

Nutrition information per serving: Kcal: 264, Protein: 7.2g, Carbs: 78.6g, Fats: 1.7g

46.   Chia Juice

Ingredients:

1 large cucumber, sliced

1 medium-sized Granny Smith's apple, cored

1 large banana, sliced

1 tbsp of chia seeds

2 oz of water

Preparation:

Wash the cucumber and cut into thick slices. Set aside.

Wash the apple and cut in half. Remove the core and cut into bite-sized pieces. Set aside.

Peel the banana and cut into thin slices. Set aside.

Now, combine cucumber, apple, and banana in a juicer and process until juiced.

Transfer to serving glasses and stir in the chia seeds.

Add few ice cubes and refrigerate for 10 minutes before serving.

Stir in the water after refrigerating and enjoy!

Nutrition information per serving: Kcal: 186, Protein: 6.2g, Carbs: 41.4g, Fats: 5g

47.   Parsnip Broccoli Juice

Ingredients:

1 cup parsnip, trimmed

1 cup fresh broccoli

1 cup honeydew melon, chopped

1 cup Brussels sprouts, trimmed

1 medium-sized Red Delicious apple, cored

2 oz water

Preparation:

Cut the honeydew melon lengthwise in half. Scoop out the seeds using a spoon. Cut one large wedge and peel it. Cut into small chunks and place in a bowl. Wrap the rest of the melon in a plastic foil and refrigerate.

Wash the Brussels sprouts and trim off the outer leaves. Cut in half and set aside.

Wash the parsnips and cut into thick slices. Fill into the measuring cup and reserve the rest for some other juice. Set aside.

Wash the broccoli and chop into small pieces. Set aside.

Wash the apple and remove the core. Cut into bite-sized pieces and set aside.

Now, combine parsnips, broccoli, melon, Brussels sprouts, and apple in a juicer. Process until juiced.

Transfer to serving glasses and stir in the water. Add some ice and serve!

Nutrition information per serving: Kcal: 251, Protein: 8.7g, Carbs: 75.1g, Fats: 1.5g

48.   Cantaloupe Radish Juice

Ingredients:

1 cup of cantaloupe, cubed

2 medium-sized radishes, trimmed

1 ginger root knob, 1-inch

2 tsp maple syrup

2 oz water

Preparation:

Cut the cantaloupe in half. Scoop out the seeds and flesh. You will need about one large wedge for one cup. Cut and peel it. Chop into chunks and set aside. Reserve the rest of the cantaloupe in a refrigerator.

Rinse the radishes and trim off the green parts. Cut into small pieces and set aside.

Peel the ginger root knob and set aside.

Combine cantaloupe, radishes, and ginger in a juicer. Transfer to serving glasses and stir in the honey and water.

Add few ice cubes or refrigerate for 5 minutes before serving.

Nutrition information per serving: Kcal: 250, Protein: 4.9g, Carbs: 74.3g, Fats: 0.8g

49.   Papaya Carrot Juice

Ingredients:

1 large papaya, seeded and peeled

2 large carrots, sliced

1 large banana, sliced

2 oz coconut water

Preparation:

Peel the papaya and cut lengthwise in half. Scoop out the black seeds and flesh using a spoon. Cut into small chunks. Set aside.

Wash the carrots and cut into thick slices. Set aside.

Peel the banana and cut into thin slices. Set aside.

Now, combine papaya, carrots, and banana in a juicer and process until juiced.

Transfer to serving glasses and stir in the coconut water. Add few ice cubes or refrigerate before serving.

Enjoy!

Nutrition information per serving: Kcal: 347, Protein: 5.2g, Carbs: 119g, Fats: 2.4g

50.   Leek Banana Juice

Ingredients:

1 cup watermelon, seeded

1 cup watercress

2 large leeks, sliced

1 large banana, sliced

1 cup beet greens, chopped

2 oz water

Preparation:

Wash the leeks and cut into 1-inch pieces. Set aside.

Peel the banana and cut into thin slices. Set aside.

Cut the watermelon lengthwise. For two cups, you will need about two large wedges. Peel and cut into chunks. Remove the seeds and set aside. Reserve the rest of the melon for some other juices.

Wash the watercress and beet greens thoroughly under cold running water and torn with hands. Set aside.

Now, combine leeks, banana, watermelon, watercress, and beet greens in a juicer and process until juiced.

Transfer to serving glasses and stir in the water. Add some ice cubes and serve immediately.

Nutrition information per serving: Kcal: 156, Protein: 5.9g, Carbs: 44.2g, Fats: 1.1g

51.   Apple Spinach Juice

Ingredients:

1 cup Granny Smith's apple, cubed

1 cup fresh spinach, chopped

1 large cucumber, sliced

1 ginger root knob, 1-inch

Preparation:

Peel the apple and cut in half. Remove the core and cut into small cubes. Fill the measuring cup and reserve the rest in the refrigerator.

Wash the spinach thoroughly under cold running water and torn with hands. Set aside.

Wash the cucumber and cut into thick slices. Set aside.

Peel the ginger root knob and set aside.

Now, combine apple, spinach, cucumber and ginger root in a juicer and process until juiced.

Transfer to serving glasses stir in the water. Refrigerate for 15 minutes before serving.

Nutrition information per serving: Kcal: 190, Protein: 13.8g, Carbs: 51.1g, Fats: 1.7g

52.   Delicata Pepper Juice

Ingredients:

1 cup of delicata squash, cubed

1 large yellow bell pepper, seeded

1 large apple, cored and chopped

1 small rosemary sprig

Preparation:

Peel the squash and cut in half. Scoop out the seeds using a spoon. Cut one large wedge and peel it. Cut into small chunks and fill the measuring cup. Reserve the rest for some other juice.

Wash the bell pepper and cut in half. Remove the seeds and cut into small slices. Set aside.

Rinse the apple and cut in half. Remove the core and cut into bite-sized pieces. Set aside.

Now, combine pumpkin, bell pepper, and apple in a juicer and process until juiced. Transfer to serving glasses and sprinkle with some rosemary to taste.

Refrigerate for 10 minutes before serving.

Enjoy!

Nutrition information per serving: Kcal: 149, Protein: 4.9g, Carbs: 44.6g, Fats: 0.7g

53.   Beet Carrot Juice

Ingredients:

1 large beet, trimmed

1 large carrot, sliced

1 cup purple cabbage, chopped

1 cup fresh spinach, chopped

1 tsp agave nectar

Preparation:

Wash the beet and trim off the green parts. Cut into small pieces and set aside.

Wash and peel the carrot. Cut into thick slices and set aside.

Rinse the cabbage and spinach thoroughly under running water using a large colander. Drain and chop into small pieces. Set aside.

Now, combine beet, carrot, cabbage, and spinach in a juicer. Process until juiced.

Transfer to serving glasses and stir in the agave nectar. Add few ice cubes and serve immediately.

Enjoy!

Nutrition information per serving: Kcal: 205, Protein: 5g, Carbs: 62.1g, Fats: 0.7g

54.   Pear Broccoli Juice

Ingredients:

1 large pear, cored

1 cup of fresh broccoli, chopped

1 medium-sized zucchini

1 cup fennel, chopped

1 small ginger root slice

Preparation:

Peel the zucchini and cut in half. Scrape out the seeds with a spoon. Cut into chunks and set aside.

Wash the pear and remove the core. Cut into small pieces and set aside.

Wash the broccoli and cut into small pieces and set aside.

Trim off the outer leaves of the fennel using a sharp knife. Cut into small pieces and fill the measuring cup. Reserve the rest in the refrigerator.

Peel the ginger root and set aside.

Now, combine zucchini, pear, broccoli, fennel, and ginger in a juicer. Process until juiced. Transfer to serving glasses and add some ice before serving.

Enjoy!

Nutrition information per serving: Kcal: 195, Protein: 8.7g, Carbs: 64.5g, Fats: 1.8g

55.   Swiss Chard Lettuce Juice

Ingredients:

1 cup Swiss chard, chopped

1 cup Iceberg lettuce, chopped

1 cup collard greens, chopped

1 cup Romaine lettuce, chopped

1 large cucumber, sliced

2 oz water

Preparation:

Combine Swiss chard, Iceberg lettuce, collard greens, and Romaine lettuce in a colander. Wash under cold running water and drain. Torn with hands and set aside.

Wash the cucumber and cut into thick slices. Set aside.

Peel the orange and divide into wedges. Set aside.

Peel the lemon and cut lengthwise in half. Set aside.

Now, combine Swiss chard, lettuce, collard greens, and cucumber in a juicer. Process until juiced.

Transfer to serving glasses and stir in the water.

Add some ice and serve immediately.

Nutrition information per serving: Kcal: 136, Protein: 7g, Carbs: 43.4g, Fats: 1.2g

56.   Apricot Carrot Juice

Ingredients:

1 cup apricots, pitted and halved

1 large carrot, sliced

1 medium-sized green apple, cored

1 tbsp liquid honey

2 oz water

Preparation:

Wash the apricots and cut in half. Remove the pits and fill the measuring cup. Reserve the rest for some other juice. Set aside.

Wash the carrot and cut into thick slices and set aside.

Wash the apple and remove the core. Cut into bite-sized pieces and set aside.

Now, combine apricots, carrot, and apple in a juicer and process until juiced.

Transfer to serving glasses and stir in the liquid honey and water.

Refrigerate for 10 minutes before serving.

Nutrition information per serving: Kcal: 243, Protein: 4.2g, Carbs: 69.3g, Fats: 1.3g

57. Radish Kale Juice

Ingredients:

1 large radish, chopped

1 cup fresh kale, chopped

1 cup beets, trimmed and chopped

1 large cucumber, sliced

Preparation:

Wash the radish and trim off the green parts. Cut into small pieces and set aside.

Wash the kale thoroughly under cold running water. Drain and torn with hands. Set aside.

Wash the beets and trim off the green parts. Chop into bite-sized pieces and set aside.

Wash the cucumber and cut into thick slices. Set aside.

Now, combine radish, kale, beets, and cucumber in a juicer and process until juiced.

Transfer to serving glasses and add some ice before serving.

Enjoy!

Nutrition information per serving: Kcal: 174, Protein: 8.8g, Carbs: 51.7g, Fats: 1.4g

ADDITIONAL TITLES FROM THIS AUTHOR

70 Effective Meal Recipes to Prevent and Solve Being Overweight: Burn Fat Fast by Using Proper Dieting and Smart Nutrition

By

Joe Correa CSN

48 Acne Solving Meal Recipes: The Fast and Natural Path to Fixing Your Acne Problems in Less Than 10 Days!

By

Joe Correa CSN

41 Alzheimer's Preventing Meal Recipes: Reduce or Eliminate Your Alzheimer's Condition in 30 Days or Less!

By

Joe Correa CSN

70 Effective Breast Cancer Meal Recipes: Prevent and Fight Breast Cancer with Smart Nutrition and Powerful Foods

By

Joe Correa CSN

www.ingramcontent.com/pod-product-compliance
Lightning Source LLC
Chambersburg PA
CBHW030257030426
42336CB00009B/411